PLEASE TAKE ME HOME
Before Dark

PLEASE TAKE ME HOME
Before Dark

ONE FAMILY'S JOURNEY WITH ALZHEIMER'S DISEASE

BILLIE PATE
WITH MARY PATE YARNELL

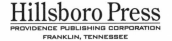

Hillsboro Press
PROVIDENCE PUBLISHING CORPORATION
FRANKLIN, TENNESSEE

Printed in the United States of America

10   09   08   07   06   1   2   3   4   5

Library of Congress Control Number: 2006937298

ISBN-13: 978-1-57736-389-7
ISBN-10: 1-57736-389-2

Cover and page design by LeAnna Massingille
Cover photo by Billie Pate

Material by Beldon C. Lane referenced or quoted on pages 4–5; 64:
Copyright 1991 *Christian Century*. Reprinted by permission from the
Aug. 21–28, 1991, issue of the *Christian Century*. Subscriptions: $49/yr.
from P.O. Box 278, Mt. Morris, IL 61054. 1-800-208-4097.

Scripture quotations marked NIV are taken from HOLY BIBLE,
NEW INTERNATIONAL VERSION®. Copyright © 1973, 1978, 1984
by International Bible Society. Used by permission of
Zondervan Publishing House.

Poems at the start of each chapter written by Billie Pate.

HILLSBORO PRESS
imprint of
Providence Publishing Corporation
238 Seaboard Lane • Franklin, Tennessee 37067
www.providence-publishing.com
800-321-5692

To Nancy and Kenneth,
our siblings who stayed in close contact with our parents
in loving day-to-day support

Contents

Appendices

Preface

Alzheimer's Patient Descent

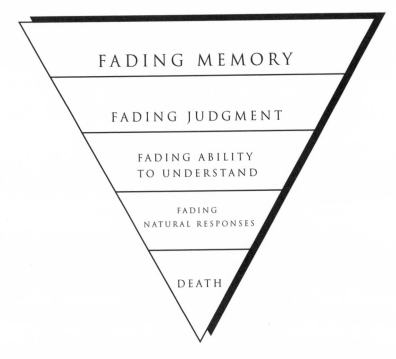

FADING MEMORY

FADING JUDGMENT

FADING ABILITY
TO UNDERSTAND

FADING
NATURAL RESPONSES

DEATH

This book is a combination of the personal and practical aspects of one family's journey with their mother, who was dying with Alzheimer's disease. Poignant illustrations, observations of change in the family's loved one, and practical suggestions to caregivers accompany a factual analysis of the progressive destruction caused by the disease.

Acknowledgments

While our mother did use the words, "Please take me home before dark," the title idea was enhanced by a prose poem, "Let Me Get Home Before Dark," by Robertson McQuilkin, former president of Columbia Bible College in Columbia, South Carolina.

The authors are two of a team of caregivers and people who consistently helped care for our mother, Hattie Pate. Others included: Kenneth and Brenda Pate, our brother and his wife; Nancy Hood and Mary Hood Oney, our sister and her daughter; Carl Yarnell, Mary's husband; church members, especially Mother's Sunday school class; friends Mary Carter, Sue Raley, Linda Lawson Still, and Myrte Veach; Elaine Dickson, a trusted and loyal friend who supported us during our journey with Mother, and who provided encouragement and technical assistance in preparing the book manuscript; live-ins, sitters, and home health personnel; and employees of Hospice, Inc., especially Edie and Helen.

The stories in this book belong to both of us, and to our siblings as well. When the storyteller is identified as "I," Billie is speaking. The identification of Mary and other speakers occurs when necessary to clarify or when the story is unique to one of the writers.

We received professional manuscript assistance from Carla Dickerson, who typed the manuscript; and also from Douglas Anderson, Karen Calhoun, Anne Davis, Elaine Dickson, Laura Kendall, Sue Raley, Linda Lawson Still, and Myrte Veach. Their insights provided encouragement and valuable feedback.

PLEASE TAKE ME HOME
Before Dark

Chapter One

THE LONGEST DAY

WHEN I FORGET,
  PLEASE REMEMBER WHO I AM:
MY LOVE FOR KITTENS AND BIRDS AND FLOWERS,
  AND MY JOY IN MAKING DRESSES FOR
  A CHILD LIVING IN A COLORLESS WORLD.

WHEN I FORGET,
  PLEASE REMEMBER
HOW MUCH I LOVE THE CHANGING OF THE SEASONS
  AND HOLIDAYS—ESPECIALLY THE WONDER
  OF CHRISTMAS.

WHEN I FORGET,
  PLEASE REMEMBER
HOW PROUD I AM OF ALL MY CHILDREN,
  AND MY COMFORT IN GOING TO CHURCH.

WHEN I FORGET,
  PLEASE REMEMBER WHO I AM,
AND HELP ME FIND AND BE MYSELF,
  AS LONG AS PART OF ME REMAINS.

The deaths of our parents were drastically different. One died swiftly and conclusively; the other lingered for more than ten years of loving care, unrelenting grief and frustration, and sometimes battles with guilt-producing impatience. The two ways of dying do not suggest more or less grief, more or less love and caring, nor more or fewer wonderful memories. They represent two sets of expectations about death and how we are prepared to cope.

Our father's death came with abruptness and finality, the result of a catastrophic, violent event in his chest. He was pronounced dead in less than twenty-four hours. Our mother, sister, and brother gathered for the night-long vigil. I was the last to arrive because of the distance I had to travel. When I entered the hospital room, three distinct images told the story: (1) the umbilical tubes and the ashen emptiness of my father's face; (2) the shock and sadness on my siblings' faces; and (3) the pathos and bewilderment on my mother's face. The way she approached his death on this night and the grief process in the months and years ahead were benchmarks of her journey with Alzheimer's disease.

Somewhat early in our experience with Alzheimer's, my pastor shared with me an article by Beldon C. Lane. At the time, Lane's mother was traveling the long road paved with the heartbreak of this disease. He used vivid imagery from both mythology and the Bible to contrast two different modes of dying and how our culture prepares us for one more than for the other. I gleaned important insights from the article that helped us along the way.[1]

On one hand, death, or the threat of certain death, comes with unexpected suddenness, sometimes with great drama. We respond with theatrical courage, even heroics. The spiritual and physical energy to cope are put in full throttle. Our subconscious assures us that if we hold on, we can quickly and effectively get through the rituals to the other side of this event. In no way does this reasoning minimize the faith required to get through, nor the grief to process during and after, such a death. The attitudes and coping skills, however, are fueled by our cultural experience.

Our society thrives on action: fixing things, solving problems, completing projects, replacing products with new and better ones, or handling issues and moving on. We imagine we can deal with death in the same way.

Nothing reminds us more of the inadequacy of some of our cultural norms or our own mortality as our inability to control how our loved ones die. I remember with haunting familiarity the words of my mother when she was still quite young: "If I ever get to the place I don't know what I'm doing, I don't want to live." Apparently we looked at her with a gentle reprimand for such thinking, because she followed with "I mean it, now." How does a son or daughter deal with such a wish of a mother? The thought is not in keeping with our spiritual values, cultural practices, nor their dying morality. So, how can we honor her wishes through the tedious, difficult death in the slow lane?

Again, the thoughts of Beldon Lane were helpful to us.[2] He suggested that such a journey does not dramatize death as perhaps expected (and even hoped for). Rather, it invites us back to simplicity and the quiet acceptance of life's predictable rhythms; our deepest and longest-lasting joys are not spectacular, but commonplace. Lane quoted the theologian Teilhard de Chardin: "Do not forget . . . that the value and interest of life is not so much to do conspicuous things . . . as to do ordinary things with the perception of their enormous value."[3] Lane saw the same idea in Jesus' admonition to His disciples not to be anxious, but to consider the quiet simplicity of wildflowers blooming and dying in the fields.[4] Practice patience.

> **Nothing reminds us more of the inadequacy of some of our cultural norms or our own mortality as our inability to control how our loved ones die.**

During our mother's extended illness, we often longed for floods of grace and mercy—an end to the rhythms of blooming and dying. But we received with gratitude the mercy drops falling quietly and consistently, enabling us to care for her. God was faithful.

Our long day's journey into night is about our mother's dying with severe dementia, the result of Alzheimer's disease. We share our stories to illustrate the progression and emotion of the disease as we experienced it. In very intimate terms, we discuss our responses and offer suggestions to any who may be entering, in the middle of, or trying to heal from similar experiences.

Since every journey is different, an exact definition of the stages of Alzheimer's is neither available nor appropriate. Our description of the process is influenced by several sources, but especially *Mayo Clinic on Alzheimer's Disease,* and *How We Die,* by Sherwin B. Nuland. The symptoms do not fall rigidly into predictable increments. They advance, regress, and overlap. The process is not a straight line between life and death. Nor is it ever the same in two individuals. But there will be touchpoints when others will feel the same type of gentleness, joy, frustrations, sadness, bondage, hope, and release that we experienced. Some will say, "I've been there"; "I am there now"; or "I know a friend who is facing this experience."

As the subtle hints of Mother's illness blended into a certain profile of Alzheimer's illness, we experienced the classic stages of grief. This was a period of extreme family stresses and some conflict. We may have been at different places in the journey initially, but when we finally faced our fears and began to accept the diagnosis, we started searching for coping tools. The search never ended. Nor did the stress on mind and body. But the need to deny, rationalize, or defeat this inevitable process diminished. We joined her in the journey. Our tasks became not to fix this egregious disease, but to accept it, to care for our mother, to preserve her dignity, and to watch intently for moments to connect with her and to experience who she was. Each time we did, we joined her on the mystery-strewn path she traveled toward her journey's end.

The day-to-day care produced weariness and deepening sadness. Days grew into months, months into years. People forgot. When they did ask, they would say, "How's your mother, about the same?" and would move quickly to another subject. We don't blame them. There were no dramatics, no heroic stories. We were simply loving our mother and, by so doing, honoring her life as we had known it. Sometimes the known way commingled with her new way of living, even as she was dying. Every day there were surprises which imprinted our lives with the eternal values in doing ordinary, inconspicuous things well. This was true, for example, when Mother's acceptance of one tiny spoonful of food was our greatest triumph of the day. She sometimes smiled knowingly when we showed such joy.

These miniscule victories brought to mind William Blake's inspirational verse:

> To see a world in a grain of sand,
>
> And a heaven in a wildflower,
>
> Hold infinity in the palm of your hand,
>
> And eternity in an hour.[5]

Even so, our sadness and loneliness grew as we watched our mother drift farther from the moorings she understood and where she had once felt safe.

When Something Goes Wrong

When family members and friends experience the painful changes taking place in a loved one, they can only make assumptions about what is happening. Each person is different, with varied genetics, medical histories, and current health challenges. Diagnosis of Alzheimer's disease and treatment options require early professional expertise.

Even as we hear the painful and unsettling news that a loved one has Alzheimer's disease, we hold to the hope for more effective treatment, if not for a cure, in the near future. Medications are available now which delay symptoms of the disease if administered early enough.

A 2005 special edition of *Newsweek* reviewed spectacular and promising research being done in the treatment of Alzheimer's and other leading causes of death. Writer Geoffrey Cowley made the bold claim that in the not-too-distant future, Alzheimer's could become as manageable as high blood pressure.[6] Of course, he pointed out conditions to this claim. Other information in this issue of *Newsweek* described research underway to discover and target "misfolded" or clustered protein molecules believed by some scientists to be the triggers of Alzheimer's disease.[7]

The clinical application of this dramatic research is in the future, and no one can predict how soon lifesaving help will be available. But breakthroughs are developing faster now, and it is extremely important to stay up-to-date on scientific research— both to bolster hope and to assure the best treatment.

Sharing the diagnosis with the patient must be done skillfully and lovingly, taking into account the degree of the disease progression as well as the loved one's personality. For example, the family should consider the patient's usual style of handling personal and health challenges and adapt accordingly. At best, news of serious illness is devastating and should be communicated in ways to make the most of the patient's skills, dignity, and involvement in legal, financial, and care decisions.

The Way She Was

As we describe our experiences with the impact of Alzheimer's on our mother, Hattie Pate, many of them are in stark contrast to the person she was prior to the onset of the disease. At least, they may be on the surface. If we listened and looked with our hearts, however, our mother was present and her core values were intact much of the time during her journey with Alzheimer's. An intuitive, spiritual connection endured. But it is important to know who she was before her mind became strewn with blackouts, disconnects, and life gaps that were too formidable to bridge.

Life had never been easy for Hattie. Even as a child, she had to develop out-of-the-ordinary coping skills. Her mother died when Hattie was ten; when her father remarried, she and her brother did not blend into the new household. Being shifted from pillar to post, including living with one family while working for another, became a character-building pattern. She worked her way through school as live-in help, doing household and child care chores.

As a teenager, she learned to sew her own clothes and ultimately became in demand as a seamstress who did beautiful work. Her caring spirit was typified in the countless hours she spent sewing for her children, grandchildren, and friends. Using inexpensive remnants, she made garments for neighborhood children who were poorer than we. She designed and sewed magnificent wedding gowns, one for Mary and one for a young woman who couldn't afford a fine dress. Her pay for tedious hours of sewing in lace and covering tiny buttons was seeing Mary happy, and for the young friend's gown—a whopping five dollars!

When she was nineteen, Mother married a hardworking farmer named Roy Pate. This was during the Great Depression, so hardships persisted. The only money crop provided bare necessities. They lost an infant son and almost lost their third child. These austere challenges, however, produced a woman of courage, patience, and unusual determination.

As a wife, Mother reflected the spirit of the beautiful, familiar description of a lifelong partner in Proverbs 31:10–31. Her commitment to "bringing her husband good . . . all the days of her life" never wavered.

This commitment did not impede her independent spirit. Our father liked her long, dark tresses, which she skillfully twisted into a lovely chignon. But during the thirties, bobbed hair was in style. So, to the neighbor's house she went, and returned with a bobbed hair makeover.

Sometimes this spirit blended with spunky determination, as it did one Saturday when Dad chose to go to the community ball game—instead of driving Mother to her dad's. That was a *big* mistake. When Dad left for the game, Mother climbed into the driver's seat of their Chevrolet coupe, got us children on board, and drove us to Grandfather's. Who needed driving lessons? This was her first adventure in driving—but by no means her last. Dad got over these incidents, and their marriage seemed stronger as Mother's self-confidence grew.

Mother's entire lifestyle was shaped by her Christian faith. Mary remembers standing at the cellar door as she churned milk into butter. Through the open kitchen window, Mary could hear Mother singing, "Oh happy day that fixed my choice on Thee, my Savior and my God." Her words got our attention; her life convinced us of who she was.

As our mother, she inspired both respect and fear. Her positive mothering came from deep within. We knew behavioral boundaries and the consequences of crossing them. Her example and her support enabled us to make good choices in the face of overwhelming pressures in growing up. She practiced tough love.

Teaching an adult Sunday school class was Mother's treasured activity. We all remember her Saturday night ritual of preparing for the next day's lesson, but our brother has his own version. When he would come home from a late date, he would stand at the door watching Mother. She would be sitting with her open Bible in her lap, often nodding, sometimes making a note on her teaching plans, but obviously waiting for his safe and timely return.

A gracious hostess, Mother cooked for visiting preachers, extended family, friends, grieving families, and church suppers. Mary has in her cupboard Mother's church-going bean bowl. Family and church members knew no one could cook green beans as tasty as Mother's—a skill we enjoyed until she could no longer cook at all.

These vignettes provide only a cursory look at our compassionate, generous, and courageous mother. She had always leaned into the winds of adversity, thereby gaining strength to combat the "outrageous fortune" of Alzheimer's disease.

Changes We Saw In Our Mother

- Forgetting recent events
- Forgetting how to get to familiar places (e.g., the home of one of her children, church)
- Forgetting to take her medicine or taking repetitive doses
- Failing to eat meals, even after having prepared them
- Forgetting to pay bills, buy groceries, or having some difficulty in doing things involving sequencing or calculation
- Failing to water or overwatering plants
- Losing weight without identifiable medical causes
- Forgetting names of longtime friends
- Avoiding social events, including gatherings of extended family
- Experiencing mild depression with loss of some initiative
- Having mild mood swings
- Showing less concern for family issues dear to her heart (e.g., a daughter's new house, a family member's surgery)

Caregiving Caplets

- Educate yourself about dementia types and their symptoms.

- Communicate as a family, including the loved one, regarding observations and changes. Any direct involvement of the one who is suffering from dementia should be done sensitively and candidly—measured always by the person's capacity to cope with serious personal information. If at all possible, avoid keeping secrets about the disease.

- Involve the person in discussions about her own care—medical, social, and personal. Consider a living will if the person is still capable of making the necessary decisions.

- Get an assessment by a qualified physician regarding condition, treatment, probable prognosis, and future possible alternatives.

- Give support to a caregiving spouse or family member; be alert to stress levels; and provide some assistance from outside the home when needed.

- Engage willing family members in required care, such as transportation, shopping, meal preparation, housecleaning, and reviewing social outlets for the caregiver and the one cared for.

- Discover community resources for present and future use as needed.

- Be honest with yourself at the outset; work with family members to develop care plans as the disease progresses.

- Communicate—verbally and nonverbally—love, acceptance, and support to the person developing dementia related to Alzheimer's disease.

- Assess financial resources available for care and the impact on care options.

Chapter Two

LENGTHENING SHADOWS

WHEN YOU FORGET WHICH ROADS
   LEAD TO PLACES YOU NEED TO GO,
WE WILL DRIVE YOU TO THESE SPECIAL PLACES
   AND TALK WITH YOU ABOUT WHY WE CAME.

WHEN YOU SEARCH FOR YOUR BELOVED—
   MONTHS AND YEARS AFTER HE HAS DIED,
WE WILL GUIDE YOUR THOUGHTS
   TO HAPPY TIMES YOU SHARED.

AND WHEN YOUR QUESTIONS BECOME
   SO REPETITIVE AND PAINFUL THAT
   ANSWERS ARE UNEASY,
WE WILL HOLD YOUR HAND
   AND BLEND OUR STRENGTH WITH
   YOUR ABIDING WARMTH.

AND THE WORLD WILL SEEM BRIGHTER
   AND MORE SECURE FOR YOU—AND US,
   AT LEAST, FOR NOW.

Memories connect us and define who we are. When we can't remember, we feel frustrated at best. At worst, we feel untethered from who we are. We lose our identity.

Who has not experienced forgetting—car keys, a birthday, paying a bill on time, or someone's name? These are frustrating and often embarrassing occurrences. But they need not sound the Alzheimer's alarm. The type, frequency, or disruptive nature of similar incidences, however, may raise flags which need a doctor's expertise. For us, a startling alarm came at least three years before we were reasonably sure Mother was afflicted with Alzheimer's disease. She left her house with her car keys and purse, but returned abruptly. The expression on her face laid bare her fear. She could not remember directions to the hairdresser's—her daughter-in-law's shop where she had gone for many years. This incident embedded hints of what would follow in the loss of memory, judgment, understanding, and natural responses.

The reality of Mother's fading memory begged for attention when our extended family gathered to celebrate an important anniversary. Several of us had traveled hundreds of miles for the event. Our parents had to travel considerably fewer miles to the gathering place. All the family had arrived except our parents. They were sometimes a bit late, so no one worried. As one hour, then two passed, we did worry. We called highway officials, hospitals, and any other emergency resource we thought might have information, to no avail.

After three hours of waiting, anxiety reached the panic state. Then Mother and Dad drove up. People were leaving the party, and some had long since left. The striking thing about our parents' arrival was their nonchalance. Questioning revealed that Dad thought Mother had telephoned to tell us they were having serious car trouble. He was shocked to learn she hadn't called. She treated the whole thing as making a mountain out of a mole hill. We were confused by her attitude, but denied its importance.

We will never know exactly what happened that day. But intuitively, we knew things were not right. What was happening to

Mother, whose first concern had always been for the peace of mind and comfort of others? Did she forget to call? Or was she confused about how to call us? (Cell phones were still an Orwellian fantasy!) Did she misjudge the seriousness of not letting us know they were safe? Whatever the cause of her behavior that day, we know now that this and many other similar incidents were indicators of the onset of Alzheimer's disease.

As Mother's memory continued to fade, we saw her losing large segments of her life. The losses were not always short-term memory. At first it seemed as if what happened most recently was more difficult for her to recall. But the loss was so much more than simply forgetting. The memories seemed to be there somewhere, but they could not be retrieved. They were floaters which sometimes emerged out of the blue and were remembered; gradually, many were carried out to sea by waves emboldened by her weakening sense of self.

When both remote and more recent memories are lost, it is as if life is reduced from both ends—past and future. In time, all that is left is the fleeting moment. The future is unimaginable. The moment is like a closing camera shutter—shut except for a tiny pinpoint of light. Fading memory is like a shadow first seen as a small replica of an object or person. Gradually the shadow is bigger than life. When dusk approaches, both the image and the shadow blend into the blackness of nightfall.

Our father was a very proud man, so at first he, as did all of us, denied that anything was wrong with Mother. When she began losing weight and looking unwell, he seemed to realize she was sick. He asked us to take pictures of them. He held her hand so gently that I knew he thought she would soon die.

Mother had to be observed closely or she would take double or even triple doses of her medicine. Sometimes she resisted bathing and other basic hygienic practices. She tried to continue teaching her Sunday school class, but couldn't remember the point of the lesson. The day she had to stop this practice of decades was heart-wrenching.

Our father became increasingly stressed and frustrated. At times he was unintentionally harsh with Mother. This pattern increased her resistance to his suggestions and ours. We sensed that the wheels were coming off, but did not override their refusal to be helped. Both Dad and Mother vehemently resisted having so-called intruders coming into their home.

At that time, we children had not accepted that at some stage, parents may need to be challenged about their independence-at-any-cost behavior. We learned, perhaps too late, that help can be provided without infringing on dignity and essential privacy.

Dad stoically continued to cover the household chores and take up the slack in what Mother lacked in cooking ability. She now burned food almost every time she tried to prepare a meal. Once there was a near-disastrous grease fire. Smoke inhalation during this incident contributed to our father's development of a lung infection with serious complications.

Dad died suddenly five months later. Alerted to the seriousness of his condition, all the family gathered. I had traveled with two friends in our Minnie Winnie RV to our father's deathbed. It was two o'clock in the morning when we arrived at the hospital. I had had a few winks of sleep en route, so I tucked in my sisters and my mother on the waiting room couches and chairs. Our brother kept a vigil near Dad's bedside. I returned to the RV. One hour later I intuitively awoke and returned to the ER waiting room just as a nurse came to say, "It is time."

I gently awakened my sisters, then Mother. Her response was my most alarming wake-up call yet:

"Aren't we a sight to travel today?"

"Mama, Daddy isn't going to make it," I said.

"You mean . . ."

"Yes," I told her. "Daddy is dying."

The look in her eyes conveyed a startling awareness that she remembered neither the drama of the evening nor our tryst with his dying through most of the night. We gathered around his bed, each child and Mother touching him as his breathing stopped. Mother instinctively bent over his lifeless figure and softly kissed him.

During the memorial events, Mother slipped in and out of a memory mode. She stood faithfully beside Daddy's casket as mourners filed by to offer comfort. She was gentle and sweet, grateful for the outpouring of support. True to her nature, she showed concern for the grief of others. She seemed more aware of happenings that day than ever again in the months and years to come. Perhaps her husband's death took a part of her identity she could not afford to lose so abruptly—not at a time when her sense of self was cloudy and already slowly diminishing.

We knew our mother could not live alone. She could no longer manage the household or the simple tasks of living. We pieced together a care plan for her that lasted seven years. The plan stayed intact, but some of the players changed often.

We employed a caregiver to live in the house and care for Mother for five days a week. Each of the four siblings cared for her one weekend a month. During these years we employed four different caregivers. Some were very attentive, responsible, and honest. Others were not.

This period was stressful for everyone. We each had heavy family and work obligations. Kenneth lived nearby and was often called by caregivers as well as doing maintenance and financial chores for Mother. At the same time he faced workplace and home challenges, children issues, and the declining health of his mother-in-law.

Nancy also lived in the area and popped in many times to calm or cheer Mother, to run errands, or to take her out for a break. Additionally, she faced workplace issues and the complex and demanding work of running a home for herself and her daughter as a single parent. She was also grieving the death of her husband a few years earlier.

Mary lived out of town, but just as we all did, she cared for Mother one weekend each month. She still had children at home, a plethora of international visitors, a pastor's wife's responsibilities, and a full-time job. The last two years of Mother's life, Mary and her husband, Carl, took her into their home.

I lived out of town as well. I had a very demanding job and made extensive trips, as Mary did, to have my weekends with Mother and to allow caregivers to have vacations. I coordinated and financed the caregiving personnel—a challenge that often plagued me with doubt about the quality and even safety of Mother's care.

Sometimes we didn't fully agree about how best to care for Mother. The stress damaged some of our roles in the workplace. Health issues for some of us loomed larger. Questions about our own vulnerability to the disease taunted us. But we all were faithful to the task—even as immediate and extended family obligations hammered our thoughts and demanded more than equal time.

At the same time, we remember those years as precious. We bonded with Mother during her process of appearing to become someone different. But throughout, her values were unusually consistent, though sometimes buried by grief and frustration. They shone through often enough, however, that we knew our mother was still with us. She was in there somewhere, and at first was often accessible. Later, she was beyond our reach.

We went through the days doing essential things, stopping as opportunities came for fun things. Mother loved her flowers. During blooming season, we walked through the yard with her, usually more than once a day. She could not remember when we last took a walk there. Everything was new again, and her joy was immense when we joined her.

All her life she had taken great pride in remembering the names of all her flowers. I would ask her their names. As her health declined, we stopped asking their names, but she would spontaneously offer a defense in case we did. She would say, "I don't know what this one is; I've never seen it before." It would usually be a common perennial she had grown in her garden for many years. We helped her by infusing the moment with an exclamation about the flower's beauty, "But isn't it beautiful?" Her simple "yes" and saddened expression belied her painful forgetting.

She watered and overwatered her indoor plants. We just let it happen—unless a small pond developed. We stood at the kitchen window and watched the birds come to the feeders. She would point and exclaim with excitement and we would chatter about them like children. I longed for her to stand at the window as she once did—clear of mind and strong—doting on her birds and flowers in the blooming months.

After supper we sat, just the two of us, and talked and looked at her book about cats. We would do this often, and each time the book would be new and fresh to her. Her responses were predictable, but comforting to me. She liked the Persian, Siamese, and Tabby. She didn't like the Sphinx because she said it "had no hair and was wrinkled and ugly." Her positive connection was with cats she had possessed, held in her lap, caressed, listened to, fed, taken to the vet, and finally tearfully buried. The connection was still there.

The peace and the positive could abruptly change. "Where's Roy?" she would ask. For a very long time we would tell her he had died.

"Why didn't someone tell me?" She looked at us through tears of betrayal. We saw in her eyes the same grief and shock of one who had just learned of the sudden death of a loved one. We finally came to understand that our dear mother was repeatedly confronting the first wave of pain felt the morning he died. In between these episodes, she forgot he was deceased. Sometimes this painful confrontation occurred five or six times a day. Finally we vowed not to tell her again, but to answer her "Where is Roy?" with a quiet, reassuring answer. We would say, "He's gone to the farm country," or "He's at the stockyard." Sometimes this helped. But she would then take up the chorus, "Why didn't he tell me where he was going?" And on it went. Our strategy now was to say the comforting thing—as long as it was congruent with her lifelong values, and his.

As she changed, we changed too. Our mother was changing in fundamental ways—sometimes abruptly, and sometimes so slowly we hardly noticed. Then the sad reality would grip us, and we knew part of her was missing, never to return. She had been such a consistent, powerful force in our lives. But now some of the trumpets that had heralded joy and peace seemed muted. Keeping hope and optimism alive often produced the sounds of one hand clapping, that is, the deafening silence of a slow separation.[1]

Mother developed an obsession with death and heaven which lasted several years. Out of the blue she would say, "What do people know who have died?" (Try answering this one!) We thought about what she might want to hear. Each time we told her that her loved ones knew she was safe and missing them and that she loved them. She would often cry and express remorse for any misdeeds she may have committed. We would affirm her goodness and her caring for others. In only minutes, this scenario would be repeated until we felt it beneficial to lead her to other thoughts. We might seek refuge in a coloring book, her book about cats, or simply ask her to talk about a loved one. Sometimes she could.

Mother's mantra through these years was words from an old hymn by William Walker. Without any obvious prompting, she would often sing her version:

> This world is not my home
>
> I'm just a' passing through . . .
>
> If heaven's not my home,
>
> O Lord, what can I do?
>
> Angels beckon me,
>
> from heaven's open door
>
> And I can't feel at home
>
> in this world anymore.

This was a poignant expression of her feelings of lonely suspension between two worlds: one she no longer understood, and one she longed for but could not enter. The task that challenged us most was to help her make connections, both with us and within her world. We needed ways to communicate, tap her remaining skills, preserve her dignity, show respect for her as an adult, and to show love and patience. We worked at this in a mixed milieu of hope and discouragement.

> **The task that challenged us most was to help her make connections both with us and within her world.**

Since each of us children was directly responsible for Mother's care for one weekend a month, we have unique stories. During warm weather, as I left to travel the long road to my home, she would stand at the end of the walk beside the driveway. I would slow nearly to a stop, lower the car window, and give her a thumbs-up. I can still recall her warm smile and her courageous thumbs-up to lift me as I traveled. I would watch her in my rearview mirror until I turned the corner onto the next street. Her image would grow smaller, then disappear—so symbolic of our journey. At first hot tears poured out of my eyes; then I began decompressing and working on reentering my other world.

At times it was difficult to be hopeful about the future. Hope continues to be reinforced, however, by advances in medical research. Even during the writing of this book, the evening news highlighted findings which could make possible the restoration of some lost memory in Alzheimer's patients. As always, this is a possibility, not a promise. Conditions include early diagnosis of the disease as well as research and development with "legs."

Changes We Saw In Our Mother

- Losing personal items and compulsively searching for them

- Forgetting most recent events

- Having difficulty naming her children unless prompted

- Showing signs of loneliness and paranoia

- Having trouble finding words or using language correctly

- Waning ability to carry on a meaningful conversation

- Losing all ability to cook and do household activities

- Showing evidence of lost connections between the past and present

- Having difficulty making simple choices

- Displaying frustration and anger about changing circumstances; for example, the "intrusion" of caregivers

- Losing retention of essential facts such as appointments, sense of time, and directions to familiar places

- Forgetting her husband had died

- Asking repetitive questions

- Requiring help with essential activities of daily living

Caregiving Caplets

- Provide help with activities of daily living, but engage the person in as many activities as possible: dressing, mouth hygiene, kitchen duties, shopping, taking medication, etc.

- Plan for social contacts that are familiar to the loved one: family gatherings, church, beauty shop visits, and shopping. Engage her or him in decisions and conversation. Communicate respect and reassurance. Be patient with insecurity in these situations; stay as relaxed as possible.

- Review and practice the communication tips in appendix C.

- Maintain a diet of familiar foods and make sure meals are taken on time.

- Avoid trying to coach the loved one into remembering people and experiences when frustration is evident. Fill in information as needed to maintain a comfort level, but do not talk for the person. Ask simple questions as prompters; be specific.

- Be present at various times throughout the day when simple experiences are genuinely shared.

- Join the person in a world of the past that no longer exists, unless there is risk of personal harm or a violation of his or her integrity.

- Avoid condescension when interacting, especially when the person is somewhat repetitive, inept, and illogical.

- Seek out community resources that can give
  both the person and the caregiver respite
  and diversion: Alzheimer's Association,
  senior citizens agencies, church and
  volunteer organizations, in-home care
  agencies, Meals-on-Wheels, care managers,
  registries of sitters and companions,
  adult day care, area agency on aging
  and disability, and others.

- Subscribe to a help line service if the
  loved one is still spending time unattended.
  This may not be practical if memory has
  seriously deteriorated.

- Face any denial, anger, and frustration you
  may feel as a caregiver; seek professional help
  should these feelings continue to mount.

Chapter Three

ECLIPSE AT NOONDAY

WHEN YOUR FAVORITE CAT DIES
   BUT YOU DO NOT REMEMBER,
WE WILL BRING YOU A LIFELIKE TABBY,
   TO CUDDLE AND TALK TO JUST THE SAME.

WHEN YOU CAN NO LONGER MAKE RATIONAL
   DECISIONS ABOUT EVERYDAY THINGS,
WE WILL BE SENSITIVE TO YOUR
   EMBARRASSMENT AND CONFUSION,
AND HELP YOU FIND AN OPTION THAT USES
   A WELL-HONED SKILL.

OUR CUES TO HELP YOU FUNCTION
   WILL BE GENTLY SPOKEN AND AS
   PRIVATE AS POSSIBLE,
BECAUSE WE SEE IN YOUR EYES
   THE PAIN AND FEAR OF YOUR SHRINKING WORLD
   AND THE ECLIPSE OF YOUR SELF-ESTEEM.

Fading judgment is a crossover point in the progression of Alzheimer's disease. As in all descriptive terms, fading judgment/ rational thought cannot be applied as a sudden phenomenon. But increasingly fading judgment, along with memory loss, moves the patient to another level. It is like watching a beautiful picture fade in a Polaroid reversal process.

Our everyday judgments and choices are based on genetics, experiences, values, rational thought, culture, and presenting circumstances. These are integrated to enable us to think rationally and to make congruent judgments consistent with who we are.

Memory loss alone may not reflect declining judgment. As such loss worsens, however, missing elements of the decision-making process begin to flaw judgments we bring to a situation. Integration gives way to disintegration. Part of what's needed to make judgments is missing or is disconnected. The reel of accumulated life pictures is broken, interrupted, or dissected. The photos fade. They have disintegrated. The question becomes not only what to call an object, but also what to do with it. We recall with unabating pathos, and sometimes humor, some of the misjudgments Mother made. Some were large; some were incidental.

Mother was committed to keeping every flower or plant thriving, or at least alive. When we prepared meals, we could find fewer and fewer cups, glasses, emptied jelly jars, and small Tupperware containers. We knew where to look. She would take a broken leaf or stem from a plant and place it in water in a small container to take root. Before her condition worsened, we would kindly tease her and recover some of the containers for necessary household use.

One night, when I had not been with her for three weeks, we were preparing for bed. She removed her dentures; I cleaned them. Then I looked for her denture caddy. When I asked her where it was, she looked frustrated. Then an idea struck me. I pulled back the curtain on the bathroom window. There it was. Her denture caddy was home now to a slimy, hopeless leaf that she could not let go. I said, "Here it is!" Her eyes brightened, then saddened. We quickly found another home for the leaf. I took her in my arms and held her close. After I tucked her in for the night, I cried.

Mother continued to ask about Roy. But her questions now reflected confused thoughts about her own father and her husband. She could not separate their experiences in areas such as occupations, travels, etc. Though we surrounded her with pictures of her husband and children, we had to help her name them. She mistook her young granddaughter for her daughter. Sometimes she did not recognize her two out-of-town children, and soon she stopped trying to call our names. She sometimes confused her son with our father and fretted when he would leave after a visit. Though in our hearts we understood, we cannot deny the deep disappointment we sometimes felt. Mary recalls how sad she felt when, after driving miles for a weekend of care, she would greet and hug Mother, and then overhear her say to the weekday caregiver, "Who is that woman?"

Some of the live-in caregivers took advantage of Mother's declining judgment. One subscribed to magazines Mother never would have chosen, yet she signed order forms for these and for items from catalogs. Products from mail order sources noted in her checkbook were never seen by us. Mother's illness and her unabashed love for people allowed her to misjudge the exploitation taking place. Perhaps the ultimate betrayal was when a caregiver told Mother that she was being underpaid; Mother wrote the caregiver a check for more than two months' work. Her deep compassion was intact. Her capacity to reason and her judgment failed her.

Through the years, Mother had sewn most of her own clothing. She was always neat and appropriate. We noticed that she began to mismatch her outfits, wear garments that were ready for disposal rather than newer ones, and wear things in conflict with her usual show-of-flesh test. She sometimes insisted on wearing beach shorts and lower-cut sleeveless tops to the grocery store. We offered substitutes, to which she usually agreed. Eventually, we privately discarded items that contributed to her confusion and incongruent behavior.

We provided suitable clothing for church events, always with matching accessories. We would help Mother choose an outfit and help her dress. She would say, "Are you sure these hose match this dress?" Reassuring her that she looked very fashionable, we would seat her, like a child, on the couch to keep her safe until we could put ourselves together for appearing in public. A periodic glance into the room assured that Mother was still safe. One day, when we looked, she wasn't there. A quick search found her in the other bedroom improving her make-up. She had used nail polish for blush.

Despite the increasing frequency of Mother's confused behavior, she would sometimes do something to remind us again who she was. Mary shares two such surprises.

Caregivers usually slept in a separate room, but during my weekends with Mother, both because I needed to be near her and for her reassurance and safety, I slept in the queen-size bed with her. She would clasp my hand or pat my arm and talk nonstop until she drifted into sleep. On one of these occasions, she touched me gently and called to my attention the need to know the Savior. Almost in a whisper she offered, "I want you to know that if there is any way I can help you, I'll be glad to." She had no idea that I was the daughter she had helped to know Christ years earlier, one she had encouraged to follow His will even to the far ends of the earth. But her words and actions that night were consistent with who she was deep inside.

During summer months, Mother enjoyed sitting on the back porch where she could enjoy a gentle breeze, watch her birds, and listen to the sounds of nature. Because of her love of flowers, on one of my weekends with her I landscaped the area just to the edge of the porch. I spot-planted flowers and filled in with pine bark chips—something Mother could really enjoy, or so I thought. Her mind took her back to the years when chips belonged near the wood pile, not near the house or in the yard. She constantly insisted that we needed to "get a broom and clean up those ol' chips." This neatnik attitude was perfectly consistent with what she remembered about lawn care in the distant past. This type of behavior may suggest, however, that her mind had stopped making and storing memories much sooner than we thought.

We tried to tap into Mother's skills and engage her in work that affirmed her usefulness. When Mother was alert enough, Mary spent many hours helping her make Christmas gifts for us: cushion covers complete with stitching and lace, pillow cases with embroidered designs, and for me, a denim and red leather stocking to hang on my mantle. When we asked her if she made these treasured gifts, she couldn't remember.

When Mother was at Nancy's home, she would deadhead all the plants and flowers, whether or not they needed it. And when Kenneth and his wife took her to see their new house under construction, she would vigorously sweep the subflooring. After all, it closely resembled the roughly hewn floors in her childhood homes.

Mother's fading judgment greatly confused what she chose to do, but her need for usefulness was still deep within her.

Mother's New Reality

Our mother had always loved cats, but her eight-year-old yellow tabby was now an almost-human companion. Callie found Mother wherever she was in the house and showered her with cat love. Mother loved her in return. I had heard that the cat was ill; but decision time came on my watch.

Throughout Callie's life we had done the things recommended to keep her healthy. Mother held her, petted her, talked to her, and fed her as long as she could remember to do so. But now, although I felt the cat was dying, I decided to make a last-ditch effort to get her well.

Even when more important things eluded Mother, she had an uncanny sense about Callie. She seemed to comprehend the need to get help for her dear pet. Mother held her cat in her lap in the car to the vet's office and in the waiting room. The attendant called Callie's name; both Mother and I went into the examining room. We placed the cat on the table. When Mother spoke to Callie she started to purr. My dear mother said, "Listen, she's singing; she must be well, so we can take her home." The vet pulled me aside and told me the cat was deathly ill and should be euthanized. I suggested to Mother that we should let the vet take care of Callie. My heart broke. I felt as if we were betraying Mother's deep trust. But she calmly said, "Okay," and we left the room. She never remembered Callie again.

> **Mother's fading judgment
> greatly confused what she chose to do,
> but her need for usefulness was still deep within her.**

Convincing proof, I suppose, that Mother's grasp on reality was slipping away came at Christmastime. We shopped and found a life-like toy cat that looked very much like Callie. In only a few days, Mother bonded with her new cat. Until her own death she petted, talked to, and loved the new pet. She sometimes reprimanded it for being so still, but she seemed to sense no distinction between her toy cat and the real one she had left on the examining table. It was bittersweet for us. Dependable judgment seemed now to be a bygone commodity.

Sometimes I took Mother to my home to give the other caregivers a break. The three-hundred-mile journey was long and tedious, and her memory about where we were going completely failed. She would ask—sometimes every five minutes—why we were staying in the car so long. Evidence was mounting that her memory and judgment about even simple things were indeed shadowy.

On one trip, we had been traveling for two hours when I observed behaviors that suggested Mother needed a restroom break. We stopped and successfully accomplished this essential activity. Then I seated her at a small table, brought her a cone of her favorite ice cream, and went to get her a cup of water. I had barely turned my back when I saw startled reactions from other customers. Quickly I looked in Mother's direction. I imagined she was bolting out the door. What I saw startled me also. Mother was stuffing her napkin into her mouth and seemed oblivious to the ice cream cone.

I was reminded again that day of the inherent goodness of people. They are generally very caring and instinctively helpful. After Mother got back on track and had eaten her ice cream, we stood to leave. Two caring customers who had observed the sad incident unobtrusively helped me get Mother into the car. Our trip continued. She was unperturbed by the experience; I was disquieted. Mother had arrived at a new place in her journey.

We arrived at my home not too long before bedtime. She asked a few questions about where she was, but seemed ready to retire for the night. As usual, I lay beside her and was rapidly drifting toward sleep when suddenly I became fully alert . . . *Mother sometimes goes to the bathroom during the night. In her home she turns to the left and proceeds to the bathroom. Should she do that here, she would fall headlong into the sunken den.* . . . I had a plan for this challenge, but it couldn't be implemented until the following day. In the meantime, what to do?

Caregivers construct adaptive measures quickly when dealing with Alzheimer's disease. My robe had a very long fabric belt. I found it and gently tied one end around Mother's wrist and the other around my gown shoulder strap. I knew I would feel a tug and awaken should Mother try to leave the bed. So we lay in the king-size bed, tethered to one another, and slept peacefully through the night. She was never aware of her decorative umbilical cord! Ironically, her personal freedom and her safety needs were now competing claims in her shrinking world.

Changes We Saw In Our Mother

- Losing ability to separate fact from fiction and the past from the present

- Losing ability to make simple choices when more than one option was presented, such as which crayon to use or what skirt to wear

- Making mistakes in judgment of both minor and major proportions

- Displaying increased anxiety and agitation by gritting teeth endlessly and other repetitive actions

- Making irrational cases for her needs or behavior

- Relinquishing accountability for her behavior and becoming almost totally dependent for activities of daily living

- Changing visual perceptions; things appeared "glimmery"

- Having difficulty reading and writing

- Losing interest and ability to participate in once-important events

- Becoming consistently unable to name her own children without prompting

- Not recognizing the functions of household and personal objects

- Moving in and out of reality

Caregiving Caplets

- Find ways to tap into the interests of the loved one. Plan activities which capture those interests: elementary sewing, coloring, reading simple books, working easy puzzles, helping make cookies, deadheading and watering flowers, taking short walks. These activities need not be long, but will break monotony and call out feelings of success and affirmation experienced in the past.

- Lower expectations for activities requiring abstract thought, calculations, and planning, such as paying bills. (As long as the loved one can sign checks, doing so would be affirming.)

- Simplify decision-making by limiting choices about what to wear, eat, etc. Engagement is still important, but suggestions are now even more essential.

- Avoid making an issue of failed judgment; instead, suggest what the next step might be.

- Stay calm as increasing displays of anger or withdrawal may develop; attempt to listen with a "third ear." For example, these displays may suggest a need for inclusion in a family activity, a smile, or a hug—a simple assurance of belonging.

- Deal with environmental safety and comfort issues: slippery floors, loose rugs, outdated electrical plugs/outlets, steps without rails, furniture in walking areas, sharp objects, space heaters, out-of-date food or medicine.

- Assist the person to talk about his or her life story, but avoid asking questions calling for factual answers. Open-ended questions will be more effective in facilitating this process; e.g., "Tell me more about your father." Facts are not the point.

- Enable access to continuing medical care for comprehensive health needs. Hearing and vision loss contribute immensely to confusion in the Alzheimer's patient. At the same time, progression of the disease may diminish the person's ability to manage hearing aids or keep up with glasses. Stay sensitive to these increasing needs.

- Select caregivers from licensed agencies and report any abuses should they occur.

- Divert, comfort, or reassure the person when talking about sad events, even if this means omitting facts. At this point in the journey, the person is frequently unable to tolerate sadness and reminders of the loss of a spouse or other loved ones.

Chapter Four

FOUR HOURS 'TIL SUNSET

WHEN YOU NO LONGER UNDERSTAND OUR LANGUAGE,
  WE WILL TRY TO GRASP YOURS,
WE WILL CHERISH THE FLEETING SIGNS OF
  KNOWING IN YOUR EYES,
YOUR SOFT SMILE TELLS US
  YOU HAVE NOT YET GONE.

WHEN YOU TRY TO TELL US SOMETHING
  AND YOU SENSE YOUR WORDS ARE WRONG,
WE WILL LISTEN WITH OUR HEARTS
  AND TRY TO HELP YOU REACH YOUR THOUGHT.

AND WHEN YOU BEG TO GO HOME,
  WE WILL HOLD YOU IN OUR ARMS
AND SEARCH FOR THE SAFE PLACE
  WHERE YOUR HEART IS.

AND WHEN YOU NO LONGER UNDERSTAND
  WHAT YOU SEE OR HEAR OR READ,
WE WILL DISCOVER WAYS
  TO BUILD BRIDGES TO YOUR NEW REALITY.

Until this phase of the disease, we had retained some ability to connect Mother with her own spoken or unspoken thoughts. We were the computer servers enabling her to be online, if only for a brief time. But understanding was slipping away.

When understanding fades, meaning diminishes, and life consists of one-dimensional experiences contained in a fleeting moment. They are not connected with what came before or what might follow. In this state, a person cannot comprehend the meaning of words being used to explain, guide, comfort, or help. The tone of the caregiver's voice, the creative use of the patient's habits, and all nonverbal cues become critical.

If we could go behind the black curtain that drops between spoken words and their hearing by an Alzheimer's patient, it would perhaps be much like living in a foreign culture. Words have little or no meaning. They convey no comprehension of the situation at hand.

We first noticed Mother's struggle with understanding when we saw her reading her greeting cards repetitively. She would use her finger to guide her across the message. Then she would look extremely stressed. Her comments or questions would explain the frustration: "I don't know why I have this paper. Can you help me?" Our explanations agitated her even more. She heard us, but our words were empty vessels. She once sat for an hour with one greeting card, reading and rereading until we mercifully guided her into another activity.

She often accompanied her attempts at reading with rhythmic gritting of her teeth that was loud enough to be heard in the next room. We tried to break this chaining effect by giving her chewing gum, a snack, or a different diversion such as a coloring book. She stopped the gritting only when she chose to. The most extreme behavior we experienced in her repetitive reading efforts was with magazine labels. She would sometimes struggle endlessly with one label until we rescued her with an acceptable change of venue.

Four Hours 'Til Sunset

The despair caused by our mother's illness began to increase in intensity. The live-in concept was becoming less effective. The caregivers' calls to us children were frequent because of almost daily episodes of her agitation and pain. They would begin around mid-afternoon. Our own fearful anticipation probably contributed to her anxiety. Onset cues were becoming clear. Mother would begin looking around furtively. She would lay aside any book, card, and even her lifelike cat, stand up, and announce, "Well, it's time for me to head home; I need to cook my daddy's supper." We would try to explain that she was in her home and that her father did not expect her. We tried every diversionary or engagement action we could imagine. Our efforts were fruitless. She could not understand. Her stress and agitation increased. We usually failed to calm her, and staying calm ourselves required extra energy because her anguish overwhelmed us. More than once she grasped our hands, led us to the door, and begged us to take her home before dark. Imagine her internal distress.

We have dissected these experiences many times. Those who study Alzheimer's disease sometimes refer to these experiences as Sundowner Syndrome. In Mother's case, these episodes lasted two to three years. Interpretations vary and efforts to explain them are strictly hypothetical. One explanation is tied to the time of day the episodes occurred. Mother was a traditional homemaker. Each afternoon she had started preparing supper for the family and tying household concerns together for the day. When she was ten years old, she did this for her own father after her mother died. The habits were deeply rooted and the sense of responsibility was urgent. These could have motivated her even when rational understanding had disappeared.

Another explanation is more subjective and dynamic. Her longing to go home may have been the association with a safe feeling, a time and a place where her role and her being were not ambiguous. She longed for home, for her safe place. She needed to get home before dark.

Whatever the medical explanation may be, these afternoon episodes became increasingly difficult for her and the caregivers. Kenneth placed chiming alarms on the doors so she could not leave the house unnoticed. These served a purpose for a while, but it became almost impossible to persuade her to return to the house after being outside. A breathing problem caused by emphysema and asthma made it challenging for her to walk even short distances. Eventually, latches were placed on the doors above her reach after a midnight escape in her nightgown. It was winter, and Mother could not find her way back into the house!

The door latches frustrated Mother. She would yank on the door and look at us with big, puzzled, pain-filled eyes. She would say, "I didn't think you would ever treat me this way." With heavy, saddened hearts, we would simply attempt to divert her attention, not always successfully. Usually we didn't try to explain the latches, because she could not comprehend our explanations.

Mary moved to Mother's home and was now the primary caregiver. Afternoon drives became the response to her pleas to go home. Sometimes Mary asked Mother for directions for these trips. After many twists, turns, and miles of travel, they would come to a dead end in the church parking lot, a friend's driveway, or back at her own home. Mother would exclaim, "Why, you brought me back to where we started!" One afternoon Mother announced, "Today I'll drive."

"Why, Mom?"

"Because you won't take me where I want to go."

Mary sadly recalls, "It was true. I wouldn't because I couldn't. I didn't know where her home was, nor did she."

Mary describes continuing efforts with helpful diversions.

Eventually even television did not calm Mama's obsessions. She could not follow dramas or appreciate a talk show. Christian programs sometimes clicked, and she would ask me to take notes on the sermons. I would, but of course she never referred to them again. Even Sunday church became frustrating. She would say, "I don't think I'll go. You know, I don't know anybody over there." After a time we stopped going.

Music therapy was helpful and had a very calming effect. Mama often went to sleep listening to hymns, even to the day of her death.

Intuitive Connections

At this juncture, I took Mother to my home for a few weeks, her last trip that far away from home and her other three children.

Verbal communication had now become almost useless. We continued to say loving things to Mother for their comforting value. But we gradually began to read some of her nonverbal cues. For example, she would be looking at a book or a card, coloring bird pictures, petting her cat, or even sleeping, when suddenly she would sit upright and start folding her lap cover. We knew she needed to go to the bathroom and needed help knowing what to do. All the explanations in the world would not help her. We tenderly led her and helped with every increment of these activities.

One of her strongholds on independence was refusing to rise from the commode after she finished her task. The most extreme bathroom experience happened one evening when we were preparing for bed. She seemed to be in a good mood; our day had been fairly smooth. She sat on the commode and took care of business, but refused to stand up. Since she outweighed me by several pounds and was determined dead weight, I could not budge her nor persuade her to move. Something about this experience convinced me that Mother's will was in its own death struggle. After an hour of unsuccessful effort, I got a pillow and lay down in the dressing area near her. She grew tired. My heart broke with empathy, even as my emotions writhed with frustration. Finally, I approached her as if we had just begun. I took her hand and said, "Let's go to bed now." She meekly inquired, "Do you know where it is?" I told her yes, then lovingly guided her to her bed.

I slept with Mother and held her hand until I knew she was asleep. She was unusually peaceful, and I sadly reached a new level of understanding, even as her understanding of all things waned. Even though Mother could not tell us things in the language she taught us as children, her indomitable spirit spoke volumes. She demonstrated in a dramatic (albeit stressful) way that her will was still alive, and it won the day. We continued to listen with a third ear to her communication cues, because we were certain she was listening to us with an intuitive ear, and we could never be sure what or how much she understood. We reached for a level of communication that would give her the peace we both seemed to feel after that painful contest in the bathroom—a plane where human bonds do not depend on spoken or written words. That plane is probably in the somewhat unexplored world of intuition.

One particular incident highlights the mysterious way Mother's intuition responded even as her other faculties failed. She had been in my home for a while, and I planned to take her home the next day. I decided not to tell her about the trip until morning. Caregivers and family can never be sure what the loved one understands nor what creates uncontrollable stress. After she fell asleep, I packed her clothes and personal articles, with the exception of things needed for her journey.

Imagine my shock when the next morning—two hours earlier than she usually awoke—I saw her standing in the family room door, clutching her pillow, her lifelike cat, and a box of Kleenex in her arms. I thought about all the signals that could have made her aware of our trip. I hadn't given any. But she knew—in the powerful intuitive sense we all have but use only minimally.

The idea of intuition is reinforced in an article by Marianne Szegedy-Maszak.[1] She wrote that nothing happens in our daily living that does not have a neural code. The codes are triggers for all brain activity outside our conscious awareness, which amounts to 95 percent. She called this process the adaptive unconscious. She further developed her thoughts with significant input from Olson Zaltman, whose studies seek to promote understanding of how the rational (conscious) and intuitive (unconscious) parts of the mind work together to influence behavior. Szegedy-Maszak concluded that the interaction between the 95 percent and the 5 percent of brain activity is a profound field of continuing study and mystery.

These ideas that helped explain that behaviors which seemed totally irrational, and which often perforated our patience, probably had their roots in our mother's subconscious reality. For example, her intense fear of being moved in a lift chair from a sitting to a standing position may have tapped into her lifelong fear of heights. But she could no longer make sense of our explanations.

While it is not productive for caregivers to attempt to analyze every behavior, it is helpful to understand that most actions perceived to be irrational and stubborn are rooted in the patient's view of reality. The linkage between the lifetime reservoir of thought and experience and current responses is blocked, twisted, or broken.

> **Behaviors which seemed totally irrational . . .**
> **probably had their roots in Mother's subconscious reality.**

We may never know the answers to the role of the adaptive unconscious in behavior of healthy persons, much less that of persons whose minds are disturbed. But the questions do impact a society's treatment of persons with Alzheimer's and other diseases and the quest to understand them, even as language and rational responses fail. As our lives with Mother slipped into a maintenance mode, her exertion of an irrational will came more often and in emotionally challenging behavior, such as refusal to move from her chair or to eat. Our longest day was quickly approaching sundown.

In late 1996, Mary's husband, Carl, required heart surgery. Mary needed to go home. Even though we had felt that an environment including familiar surroundings and people was best for Mother, we had to acknowledge that in reality, this now made no difference to her. She didn't recognize her own house, her own furniture, or her family. So Mary took Mother home with her, where she lived until her death two years later.

Each family must make its own decision about continuing care for a loved one. The demands of long-term care are almost unbearable. No single approach is suitable for every situation; family resources differ. Mary and her family chose to take Mother into their home. The rest of us recognize the burden of the enormous gift they willingly gave us. Families should review all options open to them before making such life-altering decisions. The integrity of such decisions is measured by both their effectiveness in the care of the patient and preserving the well being of the family members providing the care.

Changes We Saw In Our Mother

- Losing ability to comprehend what she read and to write a coherent note

- Experiencing extreme restlessness and agitation during Sundowner episodes

- Losing ability to understand and participate in verbal interaction

- Displaying extreme frustration with efforts to communicate

- Having difficulty with swallowing, removing dentures from her mouth, buttoning clothing, and other motor skills important to daily living

- Experiencing further changes in visual perception (not understanding trees blowing in the wind, or seeing images on the walls)

- Being totally dependent on caregivers for assistance with daily living activities

- Not recognizing her children

- Developing inability to stand or walk across a room

- Communicating through nonverbal actions

- Suffering from incontinence and constipation

- Exercising independence through stubborn and irrational responses; e.g., refusal to go to the bathroom, swallow her pills, or sit in the lift chair as it elevated her

- Napping excessively during the day, some wakefulness at night

Caregiving Caplets

- Provide almost total assistance with daily living activities.

- Relax clothing requirements to emphasize comfort in loose-fitting garments, such as warm-up suits. Don't, however, resort to dark colors if the person has been a dapper dresser!

- Assess mobility assistance needed, such as a lift chair or wheelchair.

- Reassess environmental safety questions, e.g. out-of-reach door locks to keep the wanderer safe.

- Avoid confrontation if a pill won't go down as swallowing becomes an increasing problem. Missing one dose probably will do less damage than arousal of anxiety and feelings of failure.

- Accept the need for hygienic undergarments as incontinence develops, to help the loved one feel more comfortable when in the company of others and at night.

- Learn the language of nonverbal cues. As the mastery of language lessens, the Alzheimer's patient uses nods, gestures, furtive glances, wandering, teeth-gritting, one-word utterances, outcries, and other signals to indicate emotional or physical discomfort.

- Continue positive sharing such as watching/petting household animals, looking at flowers, perusing family albums, putting together a very simple puzzle, coloring pictures, singing familiar songs, looking at

cartoons and laughing, reading from the Bible
or other favorite books, and listening to music.

- Tell stories about the children, but don't ask
  the person to add facts; if incorrect facts are
  volunteered, receive them and move on.

- Avoid forcing issues such as a bathroom break;
  a brief interlude may contribute to a
  successful second effort.

- Maintain whatever independent actions are
  possible, because they are linked directly to
  selfhood—for example, an action as simple as
  using a toothbrush.

- Recognize that stubbornness may be rooted
  in fear produced by changes in visuospatial
  perceptions.

- Revisit current caregiving practices and keep
  an open mind to changes.

Chapter Five

NIGHT FALLS

WHEN YOU CAN NO LONGER CHEW YOUR FOOD
  OR BATHE, AND YOUR NATURAL INSTINCTS
  BETRAY YOU,
WE WILL PUREE THE FOOD WE KNOW YOU LIKE,
  AND WASH YOU GENTLY WITH WARMTH
  AND SOOTHING TOUCHES.

WE KNOW YOU ARE BEYOND OUR REACH,
  BUT NOT OUR TOUCH.

AND THOUGH YOU CANNOT CALL OUR NAMES,
  WE ARE YOUR CHILDREN;
  WE SEE OUR LIKENESSES IN YOUR
  LIFE-DRENCHED EYES,
AND YOU SEE SADDENED LOVE
  IN OURS.

Mother had moved to a different home and, mentally, had descended further into darkness.

Because she couldn't remember she was our mother, her family role was lost.

Since her ability to prepare a meal, go to the store, or complete any independent act was gone, her personal freedom was lost.

Her adaptive unconscious no longer helped her know in what sequence to do things; therefore, she lost what makes a three-year-old clap her hands with glee—the capacity to dress herself.

Now that she couldn't recall the names of members of her Sunday school class, her neighbors or her children, her friendships had slipped way.

She was so often consumed and worried about needing to go home that her sense of safety was dissipating.

With only minimal and occasional use of language, her feelings of belonging and inclusion were disintegrating.

And when asked her name, because she could not give it, she seemed to have lost her self.

Being in Mary's home was the best of all worlds to enhance, even restore some of what was left of Mother. Even our best efforts could now only comfort and infuse every caring action with joy and love. But Mother was experiencing a rapid decline of both mental and physical resources.

The breakdown of her body did not occur suddenly, just as the eclipse of her mental processes had not. For decades, humans have understood that the body is an open system, with many subsystems networking properly to complete a healthy person. Indeed, as the old spiritual attests, "the ankle bone is connected to the shin bone," and so on. If one part hurts, the other parts may feel pain. Remember the jungle lion with a thorn in his paw? He suffered jangled nerves and a mean spirit as well. He hurt all over. Now we know if the mind is seriously damaged, in time the person begins to experience psychosomatic problems.

This concept of disease is amplified in an earlier referenced article by Geoffrey Cowley. He suggests that "proteins are the microscopic workhorses behind everything from respiration to cogitation."[1] This being presumed, it is understandable that grossly disturbed protein molecules in Mother's brain destroyed both her mind and her body. The distorted brain signals to all other body systems gained momentum rapidly in the last eighteen months of her life. Natural physical responses were waning—both voluntary and involuntary. Alzheimer's disease now owned her.

The afternoon urges to go home continued but were no more difficult than when she was in her own home. Other problems gradually worsened. Mother had always been a very clean person, but bath time became a momentous challenge. Mother would refuse to step into the tub, grumbling that she was not dirty. Or sometimes she would not even step into the bathroom. The shiny linoleum flooring must have looked like water to her, and she refused to step into it. She had always feared water. Perhaps now her unhealthy brain could not translate subconscious cues into rational behavior.

> We found ourselves longing for
> the outbursts of fierce independence which had
> kept her selfhood alive.

As her confusion intensified, mealtime required constant attention. Mother sometimes poured her orange juice into her cereal or dipped her applesauce into her glass of milk. At times she returned food onto her plate because she could not remember to swallow. Eventually we pureed all her food and fed her. A meal could last for hours, because Mother had a tendency to squirrel food in her mouth and not swallow. Our emotions ran both high and deep. Sometimes we struggled to maintain patience and self-control. At times holding back tears was impossible. But our feelings that Mother must eat kept us trying. Sometimes we tried too hard. We felt combative toward this unwelcome, invasive enemy, and so very tender toward its victim.

Mary shares stories of our reality checks and our arrival at a new place in Mother's final descent:

We made every effort to keep her active as long as possible. I was determined that she *would not* develop pneumonia because I let her lie flat all the time. She *would not* develop contractures because she was not exercised. Then one day, a dear friend who was also a nurse said, "Mary, you are killing your mother." I bristled and responded, "I'm taking good care of Mom."

Gently she reminded me that Mother was no longer able to walk from the den to her bedroom. It was too hard on her heart. I had to acknowledge that she had been sitting down for a rest halfway to her room. Reluctantly, I gave in. Mother spent most of the remainder of her life in a recliner in her room, or in a hospital bed when she could no longer walk from the chair to her bed. An occasional wheelchair ride to some other part of the house seemed only to disturb her.

The literature we had about Alzheimer's indicated that the progression of the disease we were observing in Mother was normal, but to us it was surreal and heartbreaking. It reached a climax when we had to accept that she had lost control of all bodily functions. Just as she had diapered us as babies, we diapered her and kept her clean. We were determined that she *would not* develop bedsores. We cleaned, we lotioned, we turned her frequently, we massaged bony prominences. As home health services and later, hospice became involved, these wonderful people joined us in this and other caring activity. And her skin remained healthy.

Even as I share these experiences, I struggle with revealing what seems to be so very personal. But these drastic changes in our mother's personality and actions were not choices made by her (if she had her way, she would have been "out of here"), but rather were the results of a possessive disease. The drastic measures we took were an effort to preserve her dignity and to keep her as comfortable as possible.

It was during this time that we had one of our most powerful and bittersweet occasions with Mother. It was winter, bitterly cold, and we were not having an especially good day. Mother was not alert and efforts to feed her breakfast were nonproductive and frustrating for both of us. Billie, on her way to the interment of a dear family member, dropped by to see Mom. She was alarmed at the situation, and passed this on to Kenneth and Nancy, encouraging them to visit soon. She believed Mama would die that day.

That afternoon they came, only to witness a totally different picture. Mother was alert and responsive. While the girls stood by her bedside offering cheerful conversation and expressions of love, Kenneth sat across the room, observing. Suddenly, Mother looked toward him and said, "That one over there doesn't love me." Quickly recognizing the totally unexpected acknowledgment of his presence, he responded, "Mom, I do!" Her response seemed almost normal. "Well, get over here and show it, then."

This was the first time in many weeks and the very last time she showed any recognition of us as her family or gave a cognitive response. It was as though God opened the windows of her mind for just a moment and gave her family a beautiful cherished memory. She lived less than a month after this.

Finding Joy in the Ordinary

At this point in our journey, we worked exceedingly hard, and our sorrow was pervasive. But our memories of this period remind us that our acceptance of Mother's final descent enabled us to experience surprising joy. It came in infinitely small and ordinary ways. But we allowed ourselves to feel the joy. Our denial and inner rage were tamed.

When Mother was sitting up in her bed, she could see the yard with its large trees, grass, birds, and flowers—things she truly loved. Oddly, however, she often "saw" large black horses and would point them out with joyous excitement. We don't know what she actually saw; perhaps they were trees bending in the wind. Could she have seen memories from a distant past running freely in the lush meadows of her mind? Or even visions of the future?

One of our favorite health care assistants, Helen, came on Sundays—just because she wanted to fix Mother up! The transformation was amazing—curled hair, makeup, polished nails, and all clean bedding. The crowning touch, however, was her Sunday gown—soft yellow, a tad low-cut, and adorned with fluffy trim. Helen called it Mother's Marilyn (Monroe) gown. When we all saw her fixed up, we would exclaim with pleasure. Mother would sometimes smile. Maybe she felt pretty.

Even though her affect was basically lost, Mother did sometimes express love. She did not distinguish one person from another, but Mary shares one of her most cherished memories.

> On one occasion Mama pulled me close to her and said, "I love you, and I want to live with you." Was she saying, "I know who you are and I'm happy to be living with you"? Though I'd like to think so, this is doubtful. Was she telling me she didn't want to die and leave me? I can't be sure. My deepest hope is that in a fleeting moment of awareness, she felt cared for and wanted to respond to a loving daughter.

Mother's spontaneous actions told us she was still a seamstress in the deep recesses of her mind. Once, she asked for the linen napkins to be cut into bias strips. (We obliged, but with a different piece of cloth!) As a seamstress, she had often measured her cloth by holding one end at her nose and extending the other end of the cloth a full arm's length to her fingertips. Bittersweet memories flooded over us as we watched her now going through the measuring motions with her bedsheets.

Hospice had become a faithful partner on our journey, assisting with Mother's care. She was receiving oxygen 24/7, except for the times she removed her nasal cannula. Early in the mornings she often removed it, wound up the long plastic tubing, and laid it lasso-style on her chest. She may have imagined herself drawing fresh water from her cistern with a rope and bucket, as she had done years before. We smiled inside when once she removed the cannula and put it neatly on her stuffed cat. Maybe she was thinking, "If this thing is good for me, perhaps it will bring some life to this dull cat."

Just Before Dark

Mother was drifting into a state of indifference and a total loss of will. Her only expressions of awareness were soft smiles when a very loving and familiar person spoke to her. This connection would quickly fade. We found ourselves longing for the outbursts of stubborn independence which had kept her selfhood alive. Her physical resources were so diminished that they could no longer support her marvelous determined spirit. She was now waiting to die.

I recall with both joy and pain her last emotional exchange with Mary and me. I was on duty with Mother. We were in Mary's home, but when I was there, Mary tried to stay in another part of the house so she could rest and tend to other tasks. But this time she was drawn to Mother's room many times during the day. She appeared in the doorway as I was feeding Mother. Teasingly I said, "There's your lazy daughter." Mother looked at me and weakly waggled her forefinger as she had when we were children. She had the utmost of wrinkled-brow disapprovals in her expression. We were stunned by this connection with reality—and with us.

Later that day, Mary popped back into the room. I was sitting in the lift chair. Mary bent over Mother's bed and said, "Mudsy, I love you." In the faintest voice "Mudsy" responded, "I . . . love you too." Just as we had competed when we were children, I ached for a piece of this attention. Standing now by her bed, I said, "Mother, I love you too." A few ticks of the clock had eclipsed the moment. She simply responded, "I . . ." The unspoken words that I knew were in her heart penetrated my being and lodged there as a comforting force forever.

That unexplainable interactive connection with Mother was our last. Nightfall was upon us.

Changes We Saw In Our Mother

- Experiencing disturbed visual perceptions

- Becoming totally incontinent

- Losing motor skills, especially the ability to stand or walk

- Being nonsensical and/or unintelligible in her speech

- Losing ability to feed herself, chew, or swallow

- Losing ability to sleep through the night

- Removing any appendages, such as oxygen tubes, Band-Aids, even clothing

- Resisting assistance essential to her health and safety, such as baths, change of clothes, bedrails, etc.

- Losing ability to swallow medication

- Displaying occasional hostile responses

- Manifesting very erratic vital signs: respiration, blood pressure, and heart rate

- Showing minimal response

- Requiring total care

Caregiving Caplets

- Emphasize comfort and basic maintenance.

- Engage the services of health care
  professionals and sitters as needed.
  Sometimes sitters are needed even in
  a care facility to meet the growing needs
  of patients.

- Monitor vital signs to assure appropriate
  administration of essential medications.

- Be very alert to caregiver stress; take
  appropriate respite actions. See
  "10 Symptoms of Caregiver Stress"
  in appendix B.

- Take measures to encourage the patient to
  eat, such as attractive presentation of food
  and specially prepared food that the patient
  has ordinarily enjoyed.

- Puree food to make swallowing easier.
  Hand-held blenders do a marvelous job. If
  artificial feeding methods are considered,
  they should be supported by medical advice
  and the patient's will (written or understood).

- Offer water frequently.

- Keep patient clean and dry.

- Massage bony prominences to enhance
  circulation and prevent skin breakdown.

- Apply skin protectant creams and lotions
  generously to dry skin and reddened
  pressure areas (Sween cream is excellent).

- Turn patient every two hours using pillows to prop into position.

- Use protective patches such as DuoDERM where skin breakdown seems imminent.

- Use glycerin or lemon swabs to clean mouth.

- Use olive oil on nostrils to help prevent overdrying from oxygen use and cannula irritation.

Chapter Six

HOME AT DAYBREAK

AS OUR JOURNEY TOGETHER ENDS,
    WE WILL BE AT YOUR SIDE THROUGH
    THE LONG NIGHT VIGIL;
WE WILL WALK WITH YOU THROUGH
    THE VALLEY OF LENGTHENING SHADOWS,
    LOVING AND COMFORTING YOU.

BUT AS YOUR JOURNEY TAKES A TURN
    ON THE ROAD WE'VE NEVER TRAVELED,
    WE MUST LET YOU GO.

THANK YOU FOR LEAVING US WITH MEMORIES TO
    MEND OUR BROKEN HEARTS—
JOY COMES IN THE MORNING,
    BECAUSE NOW YOU ARE HOME.

Mother did not make it home before dark.

So many times we had asked for grace to continue our care and our faithfulness to the task of seeing her home. During her last days, mercy drops became showers of blessings. She previously had pneumonia, but it was dormant, or at least asymptomatic. Sunday came. We dressed her in a warm, cozy gown. She had slipped into a light coma but was peaceful. Of course, she could not take food or water, but she had no cavernous bedsores, no body contortions, and no cries of pain.

We telephoned Kenneth and Nancy. They came on Monday afternoon. As I recall, we did not speak of her imminent death. But we all knew the journey had reached the last bend of the road. Before they returned home, each one stood alone by Mother's bedside for a while. We sensed they were saying good-bye.

That night, Mary said, "Let's don't bother her with all the bedtime rituals we usually go through." I agreed. We washed her body with warm soothing cloths and applied lotion and skin therapy. We gently massaged her body and gave her the medications managed by hospice. Their professionals had been so kind and helpful in the preceding months, but they did not have adequate personnel to be with us on this lonely night.

Questions assailed us regarding our administration of medicine through the night. Will it hasten her death? Is the dosage right? Is she comfortable? We each reached deep within to our faith and experience and decided to stay the course. We followed our hearts and the instructions of medical professionals.

We remember distinctly how we smoothed her gown, fluffed the pillows, softened the lights, and turned on the tape player as we had done so many times before. The subdued, comforting music eased our sadness, but the reality of the walk through the valley filled the room. Shortly after midnight, we medicated Mother again. Mary sat by Mother's bedside and held her hand, as she had much of the night. It was now nearly three o'clock in the morning.

Mother became calm after struggling some earlier. It seemed she had moved through the valley to the other side of resistance.

Mary and I lay down for a brief rest, Mary in the room with Mother. In less than an hour I heard activity and footsteps outside my door. Mary said simply, "She's gone." While we slept, Mother had found her way home in a final courageous effort. And as she did, a brisk winter dawn broke through the blackness of the longest night.

The three of us—Mary, Carl, and I—who were in the house when she slipped away stood motionless around her bed. Oddly, we felt disbelief. While death is natural, even expected, it is never routine to a loving family. From the human perspective, death brings a devastating finality to a highly significant relationship. And although our hearts were broken, joy soon began to enter the cracks and crevices where so much sorrow had resided in the decade it took our mother to die. She had finally found the home she had aspired to find.

Our emotions ran their full gamut. Mary and I felt irrational guilt for not being awake when she died. In the midst of all else we were experiencing, we felt relief—for her and for us. The traditional tenets of our faith kicked in to comfort us. Mother was in a better place; she was whole again.

In the months, even years that followed, each family member processed grief in her or his own way. For some of us, the process seemed more challenging because of the full decade we dealt with Mother's dying. The complexity of our grief engaged us in memories of the independent mother who used to be and the courageous-but-dependent person she had become.

Our feelings of unreality about Mother's death that winter morning gave way to necessary activity: calls to the family and friends, to hospice, to appropriate mortuary professionals, and to Mother's pastor. Mary and I watched as the professionals carefully, but impassionedly, moved Mother's body onto a gurney and toward the door. We followed, as if attempting to complete or extend our own long journey. We stood in the doorway. In one last caring effort Mary called out into the half-light of the chilling early dawn, "Carry her gently." Our journey with Mother was over.

The next few days were full and enriching in many ways. We finished planning and shared a memorial service in celebration of our mother's life and her courageous journey with a truly ravaging disease. (We share the components of this memorial in appendix D.)

While this brief account of our battle with Alzheimer's disease has focused largely on its progression in Mother's life, further comment on the journey seems necessary. The challenge was multidimensional: physical, emotional, spiritual, relational, familial, and financial.

After such an experience, no family is ever the same. The imprint is permanent. To some extent, the decade was parenthetical. In varying degrees we had put segments of our lives on hold.

Alzheimer's disease does not snatch a life away. It slowly erodes the beauty of memory, the confidence of wise judgment, the affirming "ah-ha" moments of understanding, and finally the control of bodily functions over which one has reigned since she was three or four years of age.

Meanwhile, a grieving family stands by and watches a loved one fade into the shadows, then into oblivion. Children are helpless, saddened, and robbed of years of precious fellowship. But standing idly by is not an option. Both committed love and accountability set our course. We did not know what the future would be like, but we were there for the duration. Candidly, we grew frustrated, sometimes angry, often weary, and intermittently tempted to take hands off. For us, that was not possible. We found the grace not to relent, the strength to walk with her through the valley, and the patience to prevail. The most formidable challenge of all was doing ordinary day-to-day things patiently and well—on a timetable controlled by a vicious reaper. There were no dramatic rescue efforts, just tenacity in our task.

Lest we leave the impression that we were the givers and Mother the taker, that was not the case. Although, as the years passed, her capacity to give diminished, she gave to us abundantly. Her gratefulness, courage, warmth, and apparent love for us often cut through the bleakness of difficult days. Her unselfish soul could

The most formidable challenge of all was doing ordinary day-to-day things patiently and well— on a timetable controlled by a vicious reaper.

not be obscured by the anguish of her disease. Her love lifted us and others who were in her presence.

The attack by Alzheimer's disease is cruel and unrelenting. If so, what hope is there for the patient and his or her family? One's faith is severely tested, but will not fail. Medical science and health care entities offer a number of assistance options. No one way is appropriate for all families. Many good skilled care facilities are available. Any family faced with decisions about a loved one's care needs to consider several possibilities and the potential impact of decisions on the entire family. Once made, decisions must be supported by the family and each one must remain loyal to the effort.

Family members faced with caring for a loved one with a terminal illness can rely on profound promises. When I was in college, we students thought it was cool (before cool was cool) to read and quote from *The Prophet* by Kahlil Gibran. One piece of wisdom has stuck with me through the years—the deeper the cavern sorrow cuts in your heart, the greater is your capacity for joy.[1] A passage from the Bible is equally comforting:

> Even though I walk
> Through the valley of the shadow of death,
> I will fear no evil,
> For you are with me.
> —Psalm 23:4 (NIV)

Years may come and go before all the crevices in our hearts are filled with joy. But we are reassured by the thought that our capacity is even greater now for this vital human emotion. We are emboldened by God's presence as we search, not for bells and whistles nor dramatic acts, but just the joy of being and the infinitude of doing ordinary things well with people we love. And we have learned something—a little something—about the process of dying and journeying on.

But what do we know about the final journey of the dying? We cannot know what imagery or abstract thoughts are part of the death experience. Literature about near-death and dying is replete with accounts of vivid images: bright lights, almost tornado-like wind funneling one's spirit through an endless tunnel, repetitive heavenward arm movements by the dying, and a profusion of similar phenomena.

One week before she died, Mother looked upward, raised her arms, and said, "Okay," in a lilting tone, as if she were assenting to a wonderful journey. Surely the subconscious beckons comfort and assurance to the dying from both life experience and one's faith.

We were enriched by another story from Beldon C. Lane. One morning during his mother's illness, he was sitting by her bedside when suddenly she announced the King was coming for her in his pickup truck. She told him the King had left his motor running, and she had time only to say good-bye. Lane's words are poignant.

> . . . After a prolonged silence, she rested her chin on her chest, dreaming of a long ride with the King. I imagine she sat with her elbow out the truck window, letting the wind catch her hair as flowers blossomed in the passing fields . . . I fully expected her to die that day, but she didn't. Yet she saw a clear promise of that which is to come. Such a wonderful image of death . . . to be fetched by the King in his pickup truck.[2]

We can only imagine what Mother's subconscious link was between her life experiences and her faith as she was dying.

One possible image springs from a happy photograph we had in our home when we were children. In it, Mother was wearing a magnificent broad-brimmed hat and was sitting proudly in our father's buggy, which had rich leather seats and red-spoked wheels. It was hitched to a spirited jet-black filly.

We can imagine that an animated version of this picture took place on the morning Mother died. She sat in the fanciful buggy. Her smile glowed with warmth, joy, and hope. Her broad-brimmed hat was in place, and her elbow rested comfortably on the back of the buggy's seat. The red spokes and brass trim glistened like burnished gold in the morning sun as the faithful filly pulled the buggy and its rider away, disappearing into the tall trees of the forest that our mother loved. Imagination now yielded to faith.

The King had indeed come for her that morning on wings of love. And He knew the way home.

Changes We Saw In Our Mother

- Experiencing slight, if any, awareness of her surroundings

- Not recognizing any person

- Drifting in and out of a light coma, then complete coma

- Losing all capacity to intake water as well as food

- Experiencing very weak pulse and shallow breathing

- Registering variable body temperature

- Ceasing of urination and bowel activity

- Perspiring and involuntary flailing of arms

- Becoming calm, then death

Caregiving Caplets

- Trust the agreements worked out earlier regarding the dying process.

- Use hospice services as needed.

- Administer prescribed medications with confidence.

- Work out logistical and memorial service plans—to the extent possible—before they are needed.

- Share feelings with family, friends, and ministers.

- Allow the grief process to work; a celebrative memorial service can help. (See appendix D for an Order of Celebration which may be adapted for your use.)

- Recognize that grieving is unique to each loved one, and the duration is quite variable. Support one another through this process.

- Take advantage of support groups and community resources to assist in the grieving and recovery process.

- Resume regular schedules and activities at a pace helpful in healing.

- Seek professional help if grieving continues unduly long and is disruptive to the resumption of regular activities.

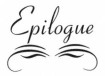

Epilogue

AFTER DAYBREAK

Our new day has dawned. What did this decade bestow or reinforce in our perceptions about life? What did we learn? How can we apply our discoveries now and in the future? Our truths and their counsel include these thoughts:

- Commitment to a loving task energizes the heart, even when the body grows weary. Look beyond tedious tasks to affirmation from a ministry of love.

- Memories made are an extended warranty to encourage and comfort in a continuing life's journey. Build memories.

- Seeing a beautiful life lived well teaches us to do everyday things with a deep perception of their value. Experience the profundity of doing ordinary things well; the big events are few and less dramatic than we sometimes imagine.

- Laying aside childish conflicts enables a family to experience the joy of unity in facing a common challenge. Maintain and build on this special bonding with family and friends.

- Understanding is more than comprehending facts, figures, and phrases. It is decoding the essence of another person by whatever means are successful. Take the risks necessary to speak the language of those who are important to us.

- Accepting with grace the skilled help of others and the support from friends calls them and us to a higher plane of human experience. Be willing to reach out, to help, and to be helped.

- Exploring the world of intuition is a natural process. It means being present to significant persons in our lives and recognizing the authority of the adaptive unconscious in our relationships. Listen with a third ear.

- Dying is indeed awesome and mysterious. But it is also natural, and it leaves those who attended the dying with a curious, but affirming sense of having been a part of an eternal event. The right to attend the dying resides in our willingness to have helped the person live; in this knowledge, we sense when and how to let go.

Appendices

Appendix A

Resources

Books

Bell, Virginia and David Troxel. *The Best Friends Approach to Alzheimer's Care*. Baltimore: Health Professions Press, Inc., 1996, 2003.

Coste, Joanne Koenig. *Learning To Speak Alzheimer's*. Boston/New York: Houghton, Mifflin Company, 2003. This book is especially helpful in understanding the progression of the disease from the patient's perspective. Exceptional caregiving ideas are presented in an understandable, succinct style. A rich list of resources is included.

Nuland, Sherwin B. *How We Die*. New York: Vintage Books, 1994.

Peterson, Ronald. *Mayo Clinic on Alzheimer's Disease*. Mayo Clinic Health Information. New York: Kensington Publishing Corporation, 2002. This book provides in-depth discussion of the current knowledge of the disease and its relationship to other forms of dementia. It also contains practical explanations of treatments and caregiving. The book is an all-in-one resource.

Internet

www.alz.org	Alzheimer's Association
www.alzstore.com	Alzheimer's Store: products relating to patient and family
www.caregiving.org	National Alliance for Caregiving
www.cfad.org	Caring from a Distance
www.eldercare.gov	Eldercare Locator
www.homemods.org	Home Renovations for the Elderly
www.medicare.gov	Center for Medicaid and Medicare Services
www.nahc.org	National Association for Homecare and Hospice
www.stbvideo.com	Videos to aid relaxation and to enhance recall skills

Appendix B

Warning Signs

10 Warning Signs of Alzheimer's Disease ©
Reprinted with permission of the Alzheimer's Association

Some change in memory is normal as we grow older, but the symptoms of Alzheimer's disease are more than simple lapses in memory.

People with Alzheimer's experience difficulties communicating, learning, thinking and reasoning—problems severe enough to have an impact on an individual's work, social activities and family life.

The Alzheimer's Association has developed a checklist of common symptoms to help you recognize the difference between normal age-related memory changes and possible warning signs of Alzheimer's disease.

There's no clear-cut line between normal changes and warning signs. It's always a good idea to check with a doctor if a person's level of function seems to be changing. The Alzheimer's Association believes that it is critical for people diagnosed with dementia and their families to receive information, care and support as early as possible.

10 Warning Signs of Alzheimer's

1. Memory loss.

Forgetting recently learned information is one of the most common early signs of dementia. A person begins to forget more often and is unable to recall the information later.

What's normal?

Forgetting names or appointments occasionally.

2. Difficulty performing familiar tasks.

People with dementia often find it hard to plan or complete everyday tasks. Individuals may lose track of the steps involved in preparing a meal, placing a telephone call, or playing a game.

What's normal?

Occasionally forgetting why you came into a room or what you planned to say.

3. Problems with language.

People with Alzheimer's disease often forget simple words or substitute unusual words, making their speech or writing hard to understand. They may be unable to find the toothbrush, for example, and instead ask for "that thing for my mouth."

What's normal?

Sometimes having trouble finding the right word.

4. Disorientation to time and place.

People with Alzheimer's disease can become lost in their own neighborhood, forget where they are and how they got there, and not know how to get back home.

What's normal?

Forgetting the day of the week or where you were going.

5. Poor or decreased judgment.

Those with Alzheimer's may dress inappropriately, wearing several layers on a warm day or little clothing in the cold. They may show poor judgment, like giving away large sums of money to telemarketers.

What's normal?

Making a questionable or debatable decision from time to time.

6. Problems with abstract thinking.

Someone with Alzheimer's disease may have unusual difficulty performing complex mental tasks, like forgetting what numbers are for and how they should be used.

What's normal?

Finding it challenging to balance a checkbook.

7. Misplacing things.

A person with Alzheimer's disease may put things in unusual places: an iron in the freezer or a wristwatch in the sugar bowl.

What's normal?

Misplacing keys or a wallet temporarily.

8. Changes in mood or behavior.

Someone with Alzheimer's disease may show rapid mood swings—from calm to tears of anger—for no apparent reason.

What's normal?

Occasionally feeling sad or moody.

9. Changes in personality.

The personalities of people with dementia can change dramatically. They may become extremely confused, suspicious, fearful or dependent on a family member.

What's normal?

People's personalities do change somewhat with age.

10. Loss of initiative.

A person with Alzheimer's disease may become very passive, sitting in front of the TV for hours, sleeping more than usual or not wanting to do usual activities.

What's normal?

Sometimes feeling weary of work or social obligations.

If you recognize any warning signs in yourself or a loved one, the Alzheimer's Association recommends consulting a doctor. Early diagnosis of Alzheimer's disease or other disorders causing dementia is an important step to getting appropriate treatment, care and support services.

Everyone forgets a name or misplaces keys occasionally. Many healthy people are less able to remember certain kinds of information as they get older.

The symptoms of Alzheimer's disease are much more severe than simple memory lapses. If you or someone you know is experiencing Alzheimer symptoms, consult a doctor.

10 Warning Signs of Caregiver Stress

Reprinted with permission of the Alzheimer's Association

1. **DENIAL** about the disease and its effects on the person who's been diagnosed.

   I know Mom's going to get better.

2. **ANGER** at the person with Alzheimer's or others: that no effective treatments or cure currently exist and that people don't understand what's going on.

   If he asks me that question one more time I'll scream.

3. **SOCIAL WITHDRAWAL** from friends and activities that once brought pleasure.

   I don't care about getting together with the neighbors anymore.

4. **ANXIETY** about facing another day and what the future holds.

   What happens when he needs more care than I can provide?

5. **DEPRESSION** begins to break your spirit and affects your ability to cope.

   I don't care anymore.

6. **EXHAUSTION** makes it nearly impossible to complete necessary daily tasks.

   I'm too tired for this.

7. **SLEEPLESSNESS** caused by a never-ending list of concerns.

   What if she wanders out of the house or falls and hurts herself?

8. **IRRITABILITY** leads to moodiness and triggers negative responses and reactions.

   Leave me alone!

9. **LACK OF CONCENTRATION** makes it difficult to perform familiar tasks.

   I was so busy, I forgot we had an appointment.

10. **HEALTH PROBLEMS** begin to take their toll, both mentally and physically.

    I can't remember the last time I felt good.

Appendix C

Tips for Enhancing Communication with People Who Have Alzheimer's Disease

Reprinted with permission of the Alzheimer's Association

- Show that you are listening and trying to understand what is being said
- Maintain eye contact
- Encourage the person to continue to express thoughts even if he or she is having difficulty
- Be careful not to interrupt
- Avoid criticizing, correcting, and arguing
- Be calm and supportive
- Use a gentle, relaxed tone of voice
- Use positive, friendly facial expressions
- Always approach the person from the front, identify yourself, and address him or her by name
- Speak slowly and clearly
- Use short, simple, and familiar words
- Break tasks and instructions into clear, simple steps
- Ask one question at a time
- Allow enough time for a response
- Avoid using pronouns and identify people by their names
- Avoid using negative statements and quizzing (e.g., "You know who that is, don't you?")
- Use nonverbal communication such as pointing and touching
- Offer assistance as needed
- Don't talk about the person as if he or she wasn't there
- Have patience, flexibility, and understanding

Appendix D

Memorial Service
in Celebration of a Life

We celebrated Mother's life with a memorial service, the organization of which is presented below. Permission is given to use or adapt it.

Order of Celebration

Comfort	Prelude, "Blessed Assurance," "Amazing Grace," "There's a Land that is Fairer than Day"
Assurance	"Because He Lives"
Hope	Responsive Reading and Prayer
Praise	"How Great Thou Art"
Encouragement	Pastoral Message
Affirmation	"Parable of Motherhood" by Temple Bailey
Beauty	Symbol of Her Legacy★
Promise	Symbol of Eternal Life★★
Petition	"Carry Her Gently"
Triumph	Processional, "Hallelujah Chorus"

★ The red rose is a symbol of Mother's appreciation of everything beautiful, a legacy we cherish. One rose is presented to each child.

★★ The lighting and burning of the candle is a symbol of eternal life, Mother's inheritance through her faith in God.

Carry Her Gently

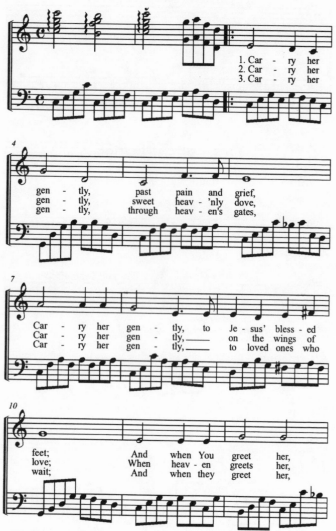

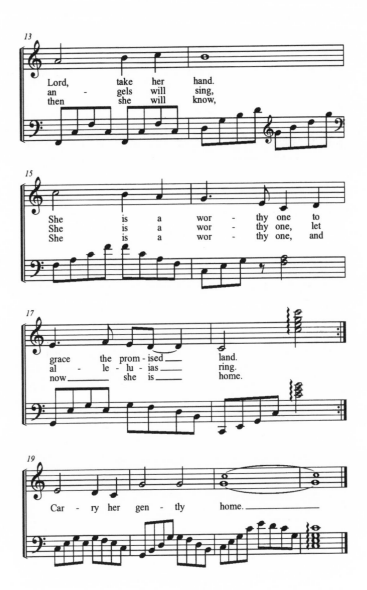

A Personal Note

I wrote "Carry her Gently" a full three years before Mother died. Her anguish about going home tormented all of us who cared for her. Perhaps the song brought hope and comfort to us as we anticipated her finding peace and safety, as well as when we celebrated her life at her memorial service.

The song has also been a part of the memorial services for mothers of three close friends: Myrte Veach, Elaine Dickson, and Linda Lawson Still.

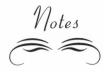

Notes

Chapter 1

1. Beldon C. Lane, "Dragons of the Ordinary: The Discomfort of Common Grace." *Christian Century* (Aug. 21, 1991): 772–75.

2. Ibid, 774.

3. Ibid.

4. Ibid.

5. William Blake, "Auguries of Innocence." *The Life of William Blake.* ed. Alexander Gilchrist, 2 vols. (London: MacMillan, 1863).

6. Geoffrey Cowley, "The Future of Medicine," *Newsweek,* Summer 2005, 9.

7. Peter T. Lansburg and Tom Fagan, "A Fix for Faulty Proteins," *Newsweek,* Summer 2005, 52.

Chapter 2

1. "What is the sound of one hand clapping?" is a much debated riddle (koan) from Eastern philosophy attributed to Hakuin Zenji, 1685–1768.

Chapter 4

1. Marianne Szegedy-Maszak, "Mysteries of the Mind," *U.S. News and World Report*, February 2005, 53–61.

Chapter 5

1. Cowley

Chapter 6

1. Kahlil Gibran, *The Prophet.* (New York: Alfred A. Knopf, 1941).

2. Lane, 774–75.

About the Authors

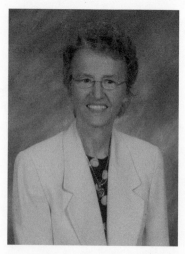

Billie Pate is a gifted writer with published works in education and music. She has master's degrees in both social work and education. Her professional experience includes writing, editing, training, and executive management in national organizations.

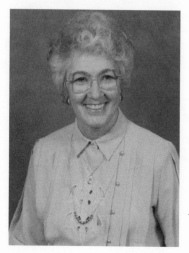

Mary Pate Yarnell is a nurturer in both her family and her profession. With her minister husband, she served several years as a missionary in Southeast Asia. More recently, she has used her postgraduate training and professional skills in administrative and caregiving functions in several skilled care facilities.